Zoltan Rona MD MSc

Supplements for Natural
Body Building

Easy-to-follow
steroid-free program

D1534496

Vancouver
Canada

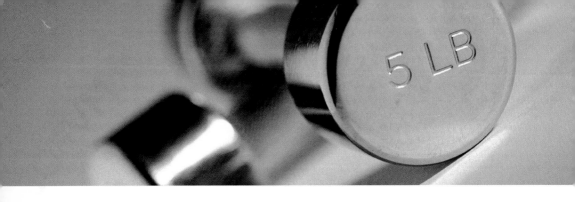

contents

Introduction 6

Why Do Bodybuilders Need Supplements? 7

Top Ten Supplements for Bodybuilding 9

    Protein 9

    Glutamine 15

    Arginine 16

    Ornithine 17

    Gamma Aminobutyric Acid 17

    Valine, Leucine and Isoleucine 18

    Creatine Monohydrate 18

    Bovine Colostrum 22

    Chrysin 24

    Tribulus Terrestris 25

Other Important Supplements for Bodybuilding 26

The Best Bodybuilding Diet 34

Conclusion 37

Note: Conversions in this book (from imperial to metric) are not exact. They have been rounded to the nearest measurement for convenience. Exact measurements are given in imperial. The recipes in this book are by no means to be taken as therapeutic. They simply promote the philosophy of both the author and alive books in relation to whole foods, health and nutrition, while incorporating the practical advice given by the author in the first section of the book.

Recipes

Banana Milkshake   40
Strawberry Milkshake   40
Hercules Breakfast   42
Mung Bean-Vegetable Soup   44
Cabbage-Sprout Salad with Walnuts   46
French Salad with Egg and Olives   48
Tuna Sandwich   50
Grilled Vegetable Wrap with Avocado   52
Tuna with Potato Gratin   54
Halibut Filet with Red Beet Salad   56
Leek Quiche with Potato Crust   58
Eggplant with Whole Wheat Spaghetti   60

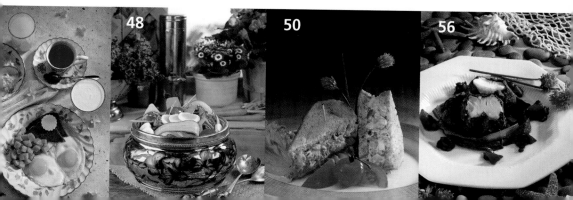

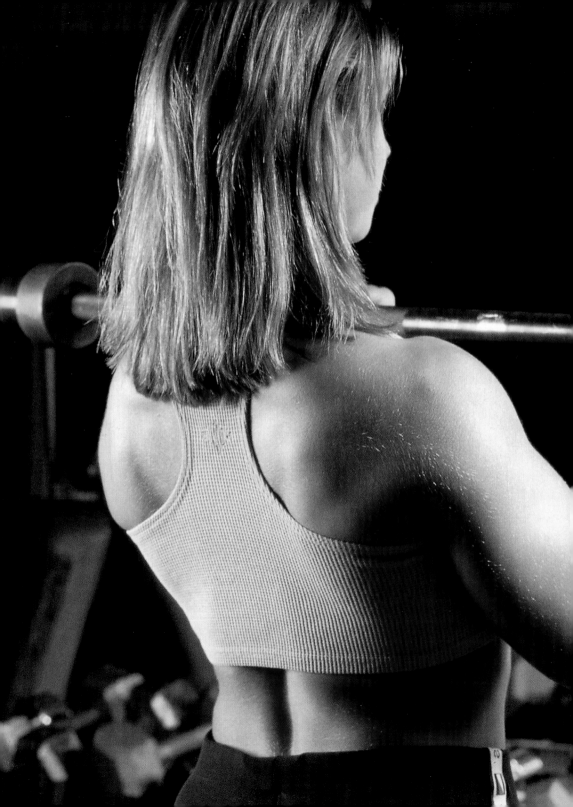

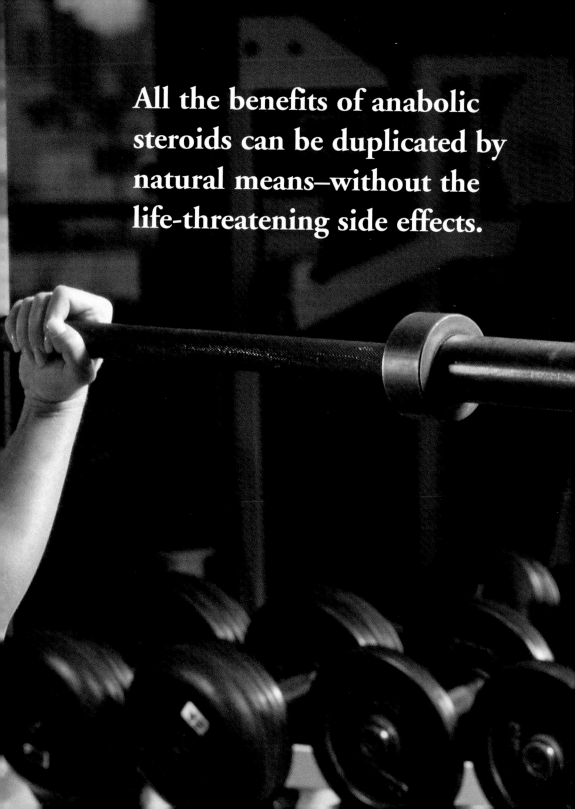

All the benefits of anabolic steroids can be duplicated by natural means–without the life-threatening side effects.

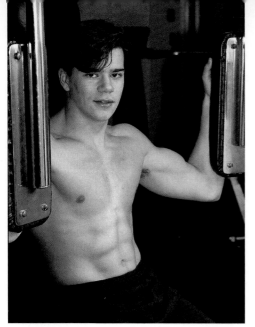

The benefits of steroids can be achieved through natural means–without dangerous side effects.

Introduction . . . .

When the average person thinks of bodybuilding, the dangers of anabolic steroids always seem to come to mind. Few people believe that the huge, pumped-up biceps, triceps and washboard stomachs of bodybuilders making the covers of muscle and some fitness magazines can be created by anything other than anabolic steroids. Even bodybuilders themselves tend to believe that these drugs are necessary to compete at the highest levels of the sport. Why else would so many weight lifters and other Olympic and professional athletes resort to the use of drugs that are banned in most competitions and are often available only on the black market?

Is the risk of using anabolic steroids really worth it? The hundreds of short- and long-term side effects of using these performance enhancers should be enough to scare most people away from using them. The most serious ones are the adverse effects on the liver and kidneys and the development of liver and prostate cancer, as well as complete inhibition of testicular function, shrunken testicles, infertility and low sperm counts. Other serious concerns include high cholesterol and blood pressure readings and behavioral or mental problems ("roid rage"). Acne, male pattern baldness and fluid retention can occur in both men and women. Excess facial hair and clitoral enlargement are frequent side effects in women.

That's the bad news. The good news is that all the benefits of anabolic steroids can be duplicated by natural means and without the life-threatening side effects. You can have big, powerful muscles and great health at the same time. It is possible. By using a healthful diet and the right supplements along with exercise to build your muscles, your whole body and overall health will benefit too. And the benefits of permanent diet changes last forever, unlike the benefits of steroids, which last only as long as you take the drug.

Bodybuilding is an activity that involves creating more muscle while losing fat. Although a quick peek at all the muscle and fitness magazines would have you believe otherwise, bodybuilding can be done to some degree of success by just about anyone at any age. You need not take anabolic steroids or end up looking tanned, oiled up and rippled like Mr. or Ms Universe to make your body leaner and stronger. While aerobic exercise and strength training are a large part of effective bodybuilding, it can be greatly enhanced by what you eat and the food supplements you take.

I am not a professional bodybuilder but I do play competitive tennis and I've had many bodybuilders consult me for nutritional advice over the years as a medical doctor. I also have personal positive experience with most of the supplements you will be reading about in this book. My younger son, Darcy, is a serious bodybuilder and is truly the picture of health. He has been following much of the advice in this book for the past several years and continues to find that nutritional supplements are a big help with his fitness and bodybuilding programs.

Some of the men and women who have consulted me over the past twenty-three years were taking various types of male hormones, mostly synthetic. The majority, however, were just interested in maximizing their lean body mass with a better diet and nutritional or herbal supplements. This book explains how anyone can build more muscle and lose fat naturally.

Anyone lifting weights for one hour, three or more times a week, requires nutritional supplements.

Why Do Bodybuilders Need Supplements? . . . .

If you do strenuous exercise regularly, healthy or not, your body's requirements for vitamins, minerals and enzymes greatly increase—well beyond the levels listed in the "recommended daily allowance." Anyone who lifts weights for the equivalent of one hour three or more times each week should take nutritional supplements on a continuous basis. At the very least, take a broad-spectrum multiple vitamin and mineral supplement.

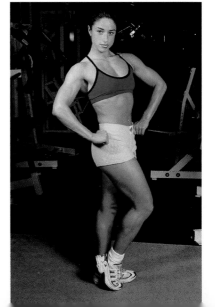

There are many reasons for this. For one thing, exercise dramatically increases the adverse effects of air pollutants on the respiratory and cardiovascular systems. In addition, strenuous exercise releases stored toxins from both fat and muscle tissues and creates more lactic acid from greater carbohydrate metabolism.

Carbon monoxide, sulfur dioxide and other chemicals in air pollution interfere with oxygen transport in the blood, irritate the lungs and create disease-causing free radicals. Free radicals are unstable molecules now linked to over sixty conditions, including cancer, heart disease, stroke, diabetes, a depressed immune system, arthritis, cataracts and premature aging.

Antioxidants and Free Radicals

Free radicals are highly reactive molecules capable of causing dramatic changes in the body including cellular structural damage and the mutation and destruction of genetic material. The damage done by free radicals is irreversible. Free radicals are increased by injury, stress, pollution, and illness. The more free radicals are formed, the more antioxidants are needed to neutralize them. Nutritional antioxidants are free-radical scavengers or neutralizers that also prevent the formation of free radicals in the first place. A healthy body will produce healthy cells—the best form of protection against free-radical damage. Sports enthusiasts of any kind need more antioxidants because of overexertion of the body.

Without supplemental antioxidant protection, heavy workouts can negatively affect health.

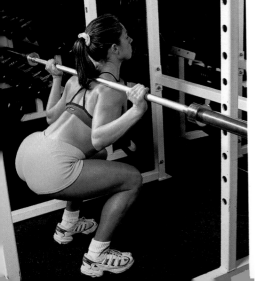

Exhaustive workouts and athletic competition can temporarily depress the immune system, decreasing the number of disease-fighting T-lymphocytes and natural killer cells. Athletes are therefore more prone to developing infections, including severely debilitating ones such as chronic fatigue syndrome. Oddly enough, without supplemental antioxidant protection, it is conceivable that regular heavy exercise could hasten death. For this reason, it is highly advisable for any bodybuilder to at least take a broad-spectrum multiple antioxidant (one to three capsules or more daily).

Such a supplement should contain at least the following nutrients: vitamins A, B complex, C and E; beta carotene; zinc; copper; manganese; selenium and N-acetylcysteine, a

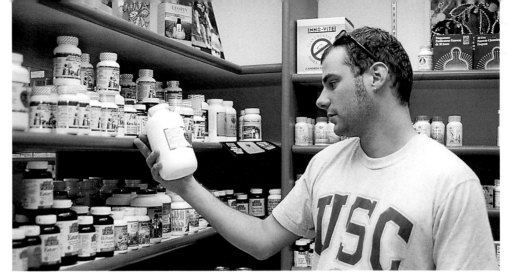

precursor for glutathione. The minerals zinc, copper and manganese are important cofactors in the body's production of superoxide dismutase, considered to be the most potent of the body's protective enzymes.

At the very least, bodybuilders should take a multi-vitamin and mineral supplement.

Top Ten Supplements for Bodybuilding . . . . . .

While several dozen different vitamin, mineral, amino acid and herbal supplements are advocated in the scientific literature for bodybuilding, in practice, one has only so much time, money, and room in the stomach! From all the many things available from a health-food store, I've made a list of the ten most important and effective bodybuilding supplements.

Most of these supplements can be taken in powder, capsule or liquid form to avoid taking handfuls of pills. All are generally regarded as safe, but some can cause certain problems; these are discussed in each section. If you have a medical condition or are concerned about dosages or other issues, consult a naturopath or medical doctor familiar with natural remedies.

Here, then, are the ten supplements I would recommend for anyone wanting to build muscle and burn fat.

1. Protein

One gram of protein per pound of lean mass or more daily is required for maximum muscle strength and growth, as well as to prevent muscle deterioration and loss of lean body mass to energy requirements. It is most natural to get your protein from real food rather than from supplements. In that respect, the highest-quality proteins, in descending order of quality based on amino acid composition, are:

- lactalbumin (from hydrolyzed whey protein concentrate)
- egg albumin (from egg white)
- meat, fish, and poultry
- casein (from milk)
- soy protein
- vegetable protein (half the muscle-building protein quality of lactalbumin).

Protein is primarily used in bodybuilding to optimize lean tissue health and mass, boost metabolism, maximize fat loss, minimize recovery time and muscle soreness, boost immune function and help prevent muscle and bone damage consequent to weight training. Protein is effective in increasing muscle strength and size while preventing the muscle tissue breakdown that can occur during strenuous exercise. Exercise increases muscle protein turnover rate and much greater amounts are needed for this, as well as for tissue repair and muscle growth. An insufficient protein intake can lead to excessive muscle breakdown, the opposite of what you want as a bodybuilder. When bodybuilding, what you want to do is keep the body in a positive nitrogen balance necessary for new growth and repair.

Bodybuilders need extra protein for muscle strength and growth, and to prevent muscle deterioration and loss of lean body mass.

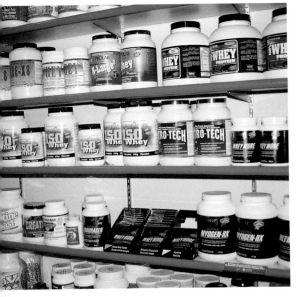

Whey, a by-product of cheese making, contains carbohydrates including lactose; minerals including calcium; proteins including alpha-lactalbumin, beta-lactoglobulin, lactoferrin and serum and albumin lysozyme; and immunoglobulins A, G and M. Whey contains a very high concentration of branched-chain amino acids (valine, leucine and isoleucine). These are the first amino acids used up by muscles during exercise, so you need to have a lot of them available for burning.

In its natural form, whey is a syrupy-sweet liquid because of the large amounts of the milk sugar lactose that it contains. Whey protein is highly digestible and contains a higher-quality amino acid profile than does egg white. Several companies manufacture high-quality whey protein without the lactose, fat, and cholesterol normally present in whole milk and cheese. The technical term used to describe how pure whey protein is extracted from dairy products is "ion-exchange." The ion-exchange process involves using an electrostatic separation process, which yields the purest whey protein formulation minus casein, lactose and other dairy ingredients.

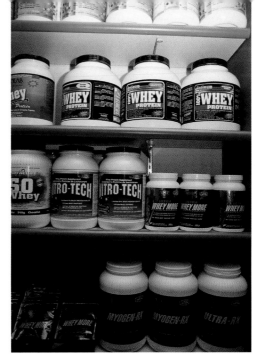

Whey protein is highly digestible and contains a high-quality amino acid profile.

Aside from its bodybuilding properties, whey protein is used as an alternative to milk for people with lactose intolerance, milk protein allergy, asthma, high cholesterol or obesity and for replacing or supplementing milk-based infant formulas. There is evidence that whey protein can prevent cancer of the colon and breast as well as the weight loss that occurs with all kinds of cancer. In people with HIV disease (AIDS), whey protein increases body weight, elevates the important antioxidant glutathione, increases albumin and white blood cell counts, and reduces diarrhea.

Individuals allergic to milk products should avoid using whey protein and substitute egg white or soy protein as a high-quality protein supplement. People who are allergic to milk are usually sensitive to the casein, not whey protein in milk. For those with lactose intolerance, whey protein powders are available without lactose. Both lactose and casein can be extracted from whey protein powders, rendering the product suitable for most people with milk allergy. Having said all this, it is still possible that some people are allergic to whey protein itself. Such individuals would therefore have to switch to another high protein source.

More on Amino Acids

Life is not possible without a healthy amount of amino acids in the body. Amino acids can best be defined as the building blocks

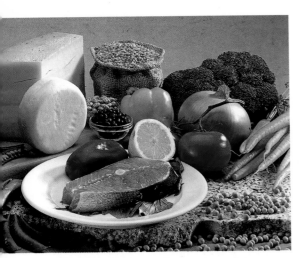

Amino acids, which are the building blocks to protein, come from protein-rich food sources.

of proteins needed to create cells, enzymes and hormones; repair damaged tissues and organs; make antibodies against invading bacteria and viruses; and build nucleoproteins (RNA and DNA). Amino acids are also involved in carrying oxygen throughout the body and are crucial for optimal muscle activity.

Amino acids come from protein-rich sources such as meat, fish and dairy products, and from vegetables such as legumes, peas and whole grains. Amino acids are classified either as essential or nonessential. The eight essential amino acids are the ones that cannot be made in the body from other amino acids and must be supplied by the diet. These are leucine, isoleucine, valine (which together comprise the branched-chain amino acids), methionine, lysine, threonine, phenylalanine and tryptophan. The rest are nonessential (meaning they can be manufactured by the body from other nutrients) provided that overall nutrition is adequate. High doses of certain nonessential amino acids are useful in the treatment of a long list of both acute and chronic ailments and are very important as bodybuilding supplements.

Some health-care practitioners argue that using single amino acid therapies is unnatural and does nothing to really heal the individual as a whole. Others point to toxicity problems as well as the potential creation of new deficiencies by unbalancing other amino acids if only one is taken. Such healers prefer to make use of whole-food concentrates such as enzymes, herbs and glandular extracts. There is merit to this philosophy, but any large-dose amino acid supplementation can always be balanced by either one of the protein sources mentioned earlier or by a multiple free-form amino acid supplement.

Single amino acid therapies can be used with a much greater degree of safety than any prescription or over-the-counter drug and, if used as part of a comprehensive nutritional therapy program, balance with other nutrients in the body can be maintained. True toxicity with uncontaminated single amino acid therapies has rarely, if ever, been adequately documented. Recent deaths from the use of genetically engineered, contaminated tryptophan (causing eosinophilic myalgia syndrome) were not the result of the amino acid but of a shoddy manufacturing process.

Single amino acid therapies fulfill two important principles of complementary medicine:

1. In the practice of healing it is usually wise to imitate the body's natural healing mechanisms. For example, if you cannot digest high-protein foods, consuming dietary substances (such as stomach bitters, betaine and pepsin or apple cider vinegar) that help dissolve peptide bonds will allow your body to absorb and utilize the nutrients from protein.

2. If a drug can bring about the act of medical healing, a nutrient with less toxicity can be substituted to perform the same act. Examples of this are the uses of feverfew, ginger root, niacin, guarana, devil's claw, D,L-phenylalanine, tryptophan and/or gamma aminobutyric acid (GABA) in the treatment of migraine headaches. Another important example is the use of magnesium as a nontoxic calcium channel blocker for heart disease. In bodybuilding, synthetic anabolic steroids can be mimicked in a much healthier manner by using one or more of the amino acids and natural anabolic supplements discussed in this book.

Amino acids are organic molecules that are the basic building blocks that make up protein. Hook together any number of amino acids and you get large molecules known biochemically by the name "peptides." Many peptides linked together are known as polypeptides and when you link polypeptides with one another you get protein. The digestion process in the stomach and small intestines breaks down dietary proteins to peptides and amino acids through a process called hydrolyzation. The individual amino acids are then absorbed into the bloodstream, where they travel to various tissues and organs

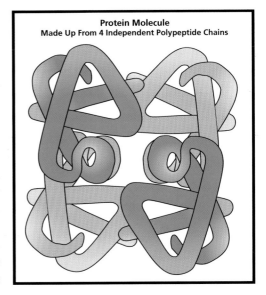

Protein Molecule
Made Up From 4 Independent Polypeptide Chains

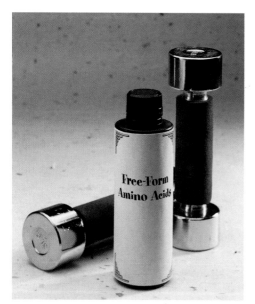

Free-form amino acids are readily absorbed in the body.

to link up with other amino acids to make structural proteins, hormones, and enzymes.

All the amino acids have specific functions in the body independent of their role in creating protein. For example, the body uses some, such as carnitine, for transporting fats into cells for energy. Others, such as arginine, can stimulate the pituitary gland in the brain to secrete growth hormone, which is involved in developing lean muscle tissue and in burning fat.

Why take individual amino acids, such as glutamine, discussed below, in addition to whey protein or other high-protein sources? One of the reasons why food sources of protein can be undesirable for many bodybuilders is that many high-protein foods also tend be high in fat. In addition, as we grow older the level of digestive enzymes tends to decrease, thus impairing our ability to efficiently absorb individual amino acids from food. If you want to build healthier muscle more quickly, meals that present an incomplete amino acid profile to the bloodstream will be of only marginal use to the muscle-building process.

The best amino acid supplements you can use are the free-form amino acids because these have been hydrolyzed already and are ready to be absorbed. Since insulin is required to transport amino acids to muscle cells, take these supplements with a little fruit juice or a carbohydrate snack because fruits, and carbohydrates in general, induce insulin release.

Despite the fact that each and every one of the amino acids discussed in this book can be found in varying degrees in every cell of the human body, single amino acids are prohibited from being sold to the Canadian public (with the exception of tryptophan, which is available at inflated prices with a doctor's prescription). Canadian physicians, naturopaths, chiropractors, dentists and other health professionals wishing to sell amino acids in their practices to their patients are prohibited from so doing. Any Canadian, however, can legally order amino acids from the United States for personal use in Canada.

Note: Unless otherwise indicated, all amino acids referred to here are the L-form (for example, L-tryptophan). The D-form, except in special circumstances, has no beneficial effects. In the case of some amino acids (for example, D-carnitine), the D-form could actually be toxic. Make sure the supplement you buy specifies the L-form.

2. Glutamine (L-glutamine)

Take 6,000 to 18,000 milligrams daily in powder or capsule form after workouts or before bed. This is the most important amino acid for bodybuilders. Glutamine is the most abundant amino acid in the body and makes up more than 50 percent of the amino acids found in muscle cells. Stress and exercise increase the body's demand for glutamine. Studies have shown that supplementing glutamine can prevent muscle wasting. Intense weight training has been shown to uniformly decrease glutamine levels by 50 percent, and it takes several hours for levels to return to normal. Low glutamine levels impair the immune system and increase susceptibility to infection.

Glutamine is produced primarily in skeletal muscle. Its mechanism of action is to work as an inter-organ nitrogen and carbon transporter. Glutamine is traditionally classified as a nonessential amino acid because it can be made in the body from other amino acids. Regardless of this classification, glutamine is essential for maintaining intestinal function, immune response and amino acid stability during times of severe stress or greater physical activity; that's why it's essential for bodybuilders. Glutamine is an important metabolic fuel for white blood cells, fibroblasts (cells involved in tissue repair and healing) and enterocytes (cells lining the

Glutamine is the most important amino acid for bodybuilders, because it makes up for more than half of the amino acids in muscle cells.

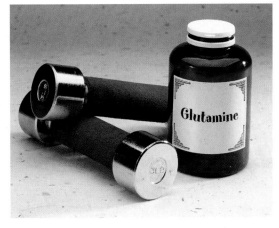

gastrointestinal tract). Glutamine also functions as a precursor of other amino acids, glucose (blood sugar), purines, DNA and RNA, and glutathione, one of the body's most important self-generated antioxidants.

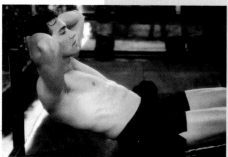

Glutamine has been shown to enhance stamina and exercise performance. The usual aches and pains we feel after heavy exercise are significantly reduced by regular use of this supplement. But its usefulness is certainly not limited to bodybuilding. Glutamine can also be used to treat the following:

- hypoglycemia
- peptic ulcers and ulcerative colitis
- depression, moodiness, poor memory, irritability, anxiety, schizophrenia and senility
- insomnia
- short bowel syndrome and Crohn's disease
- cystinuria
- sickle cell anemia
- poor recovery after bone marrow transplant
- alcohol withdrawal and alcohol poisoning

Studies show that glutamine is well tolerated and without side effects in doses of up to forty grams per day.

3. Arginine (L-arginine)

Arginine, at 6,000 to 12,000 milligrams daily, is another effective amino acid supplement that should merit top consideration by all bodybuilders. It is good for improving athletic performance of just about any kind. Arginine is an essential amino acid necessary for protein synthesis. It works by stimulating the release of pro-lactin, glucagon, insulin, and growth hormone; growth hormone helps reduce fat, improves healing, and increases muscle mass. The body uses arginine as a base for making nitric oxide, a chemical that relaxes the muscles in the walls of arteries and thereby increases blood flow and tissue oxygenation. Arginine also has ammonia-reducing effects, and since ammonia levels increase with physical activity, bodybuilders need to ensure it is removed from their systems.

Studies have shown that arginine improves immune responses to bacteria, viruses and tumor cells and promotes wound healing and regeneration of the liver; it is considered crucial for optimal muscle growth and tissue repair. Arginine is a precursor for collagen synthesis, which is important for wound healing. It is also a precursor in creatine production; creatine combines with phosphate to become an important energy source.

Other well-documented beneficial effects of arginine are vasodilation (widening of the diameter) of peripheral and coronary blood vessels. Topically, arginine can be used as an aid in wound healing, for treating cold hands and feet and for erectile dysfunction and male impotence. Food sources of arginine include protein-rich foods, nuts, corn, gelatin, carob, brown rice, oats, sunflower seeds, sesame seeds, peas, wheat, raisins, eggs, and brewer's yeast.

The essential amino acid arginine, which is found in foods such as those below, is necessary for protein synthesis.

4. Ornithine (L-ornithine)

Take 3,000 to 6,000 milligrams daily. Like arginine, this amino acid stimulates the release of growth hormone, which increases muscle mass while decreasing the amount of body fat. Ornithine boosts the immune system and promotes healthy liver function and liver regeneration by detoxifying ammonia. Ornithine is used for bodybuilding and for improving athletic performance and wound healing. It is a nonessential amino acid produced in the body from arginine; it does not occur in proteins.

5. Gamma Aminobutyric Acid (GABA)

Take 3,000 to 6,000 milligrams daily with food. GABA is an amino acid classified as a neurotransmitter, a substance that sends nerve impulses

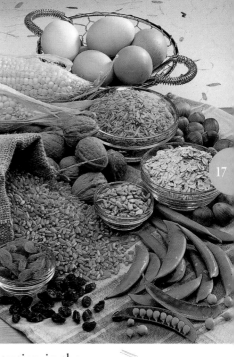

from one nerve cell to another. Its highest concentration in the body is in the hypothalamus, a region of the back of the brain that regulates sleep cycles, body temperature and the activity of the pituitary gland, the master endocrine gland affecting all hormonal functions of the body. One of the most important pituitary hormones to the bodybuilder is growth hormone, which is responsible for building healthy muscle while ridding the body of excess fat. GABA boosts growth hormone levels significantly

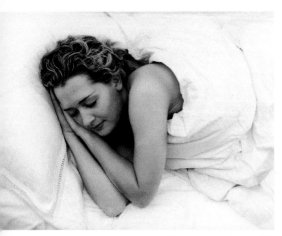

(about five-fold within ninety minutes of supplementation) if taken before bed. It also facilitates sleep and has a calming effect on the anxious or jittery mind, a most beneficial result if you're in competition. GABA has been known to suppress the appetite, so make sure you're eating all you need for your muscle-building program.

While real growth hormone is available only by prescription, costs up to $15,000 for a year's supply, and must be injected, GABA's growth hormone elevating effects cost about fifty cents a day and rival those of potent pharmaceutical compounds.

The amino acid GABA **helps build healthy muscle and encourages restful sleep.**

6. Valine, Leucine and Isoleucine

Take 1,500 to 6,000 milligrams of leucine and 800 to 3,000 milligrams of valine and isoleucine daily in divided doses. Valine, leucine and isoleucine are usually called the branched-chain amino acids because of their common chemical structure; they make up 35 percent of the amino acid content of muscle. Found in proteins, they are important for mental vigor, alertness, blood sugar control, muscle coordination, muscle damage repair and calm emotions, all of which are important to serious bodybuilders. Isoleucine is especially essential to the formation of hemoglobin, and leucine promotes the release of growth hormone. Make sure your branched-chain amino acid supplement contains more leucine than valine and isoleucine because the body uses leucine more quickly than the other two.

7. Creatine Monohydrate

Creatine monohydrate is the supplement on the minds of all athletes, bodybuilders and even those with a chronic muscle illness of one kind or another. Never has so much been said by so many in the mainstream media about a nutritional supplement than it has about creatine monohydrate. Wrongly associated with banned steroid muscle builders, creatine monohydrate has been the victim of much unwarranted criticism, moralizing and political debate.

First of all, creatine monohydrate is not a steroid, nor is it some sort of evil drug. Creatine monohydrate is found normally in the body. As a supplement, it is a natural, tasteless and safe nutrient found in animal protein (about five grams per kilogram of steak, salmon, tuna, lobster or lamb). Approximately 0.5 percent of the weight of high-protein foods such as steak is made up of creatine, but some of it is lost to cooking because creatine is very sensitive to high temperatures.

Grams of Creatine per Kilogram of Food	
Herring	6.5-10
Pork	5.0
Beef	4.5
Salmon	4.5
Tuna	4.0
Cod	3.0
Milk	0.1

The March 2000 issue of *Medicine and Science in Sports and Exercise* contained two studies suggesting that well-trained athletes who took creatine monohydrate performed better. One study looked at sprinters who improved their speed over 15 meters by .03 seconds, enough to make a big difference at the end of a race. The other study on bicyclists showed that creatine supplementation enhanced the ability to use oxygen.

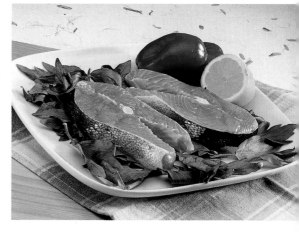

Salmon is a good food source of creatine.

Contrary to popular belief, creatine is not banned by the International Olympic Committee, the National Collegiate Athletic Association or professional sports leagues. Creatine use is widespread among professional and amateur athletes and has been reported to be used by high-profile professional baseball and football players. The annual consumption of creatine in the United States alone is estimated to exceed four million kilograms per year and growing.

Creatine monohydrate has many bodybuilding benefits.

Next to carbohydrates, creatine monohydrate is the most extensively studied energy-producing nutrient. More than eighty original research articles on creatine supplementation published in journals show that creatine supplementation increases strength, power, muscle mass and athletic performance significantly.

Creatine monohydrate has many bodybuilding and performance-enhancing benefits, including the ability to create more powerful muscle contractions, faster muscle recovery, increased lean weight gain and increased muscle size. Creatine has also been used to treat heart failure, neuromuscular disease such as muscular dystrophy and mitochondrial diseases such as fibromyalgia and chronic fatigue syndrome. It is also used to slow the progression of amyotrophic lateral sclerosis (ALS or Lou Gehrig's disease), Huntington's disease and Parkinson's disease.

Creatine is an essential, naturally occurring nutrient found in the body.

Creatine is an essential, naturally occurring nutrient found in the human body and plays a vital role in producing the energy needed for muscle contractions, particularly in movements that are quick and explosive in nature. Creatine appears to be more effective for repeated maximal energy bursts than for single event performance. Acute creatine loading might be more effective than ongoing use. Approximately 95 percent of it is found in skeletal muscle with the remainder scattered throughout the rest

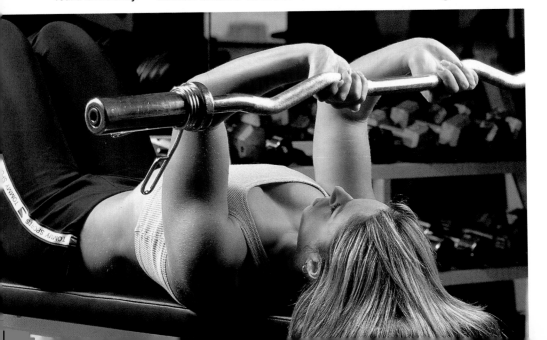

of the body, with the highest concentrations in the heart, brain and testes.

Creatine monohydrate has adenosine triphosphate-enhancing effects that dramatically increase muscle strength. Adenosine triphosphate is important in the building of new tissues, nerve transmission, blood circulation, digestion, gland secretions and muscle contraction. It is formed in the body and all its functions are crucial for optimal bodybuilding.

Creatine monohydrate is especially popular with competitive bodybuilders because it can cause them to look about five to ten pounds more muscular. This is because creatine attracts water into the muscles. This should not be confused with the bloating and fluid retention caused by allergies, congested organs or other suboptimal states of health in which the fluid accumulation is outside the muscles.

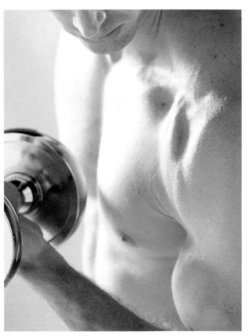

Creatine can dramatically increase muscle strength and size.

Creatine monohydrate converts in the body to creatine phosphate, which supplies energy to muscles, providing greater strength and stamina. The more creatine stored in muscles the more energy is available to activate the muscle tissue. Creatine also acts as a buffer against the buildup of lactic acid and neutralizes the free radicals produced by heavy exercise.

The human body replaces creatine lost throughout the day in physical activity through both internal synthesis in the liver from the amino acids arginine, glycine and methionine, and through dietary intake. With heavy exercise, the body may not be able to make enough to prevent muscle fatigue and pain caused by lactic acid buildup. Creatine supplementation would certainly prevent this and create greater stamina, especially in activities such as weight lifting used by many different types of athletes, including bodybuilders.

Creatine supplementation can also significantly reduce the ammonia level in the blood. Ammonia is a toxic by-product of energy metabolism that increases rapidly when adenosine triphosphate becomes depleted. Ammonia can also build up if protein is not fully utilized. One of the drawbacks of supplementing huge amounts of protein for bodybuilding is the unwanted increase in ammonia levels in the blood caused by the body's inability to use all the protein. Creatine supplementation can help the body get rid of excess ammonia and may be very valuable not only in bodybuilding but in numerous medical conditions involving diseased muscles where the ammonia buildup affects muscle function.

Side Effects

Adverse reactions to creatine supplementation when used as directed are extremely rare. With literally millions of North Americans now using the product, there have never been any deaths or serious illnesses reported as a result of taking it. In a minority of individuals, creatine use can cause muscle cramping, gastrointestinal pain, nausea and diarrhea with subsequent dehydration. There have been some reports of creatine causing mild kidney problems (inflammation), possibly secondary to dehydration, but true kidney toxicity has yet to be reported. You can avoid these potential side effects by making sure that you take liberal amounts of water with athletic activity. However, creatine should be avoided by people with pre-existing kidney disease or by people with diseases such as diabetes that increase the risk for kidney dysfunction. Check with your health-care provider before starting supplementation.

The correct way to use creatine is to take twenty grams per day (or 0.3 grams per kilogram of body weight) for five days followed by a maintenance dose of two grams (or 0.03 grams per kilogram of body weight) daily. Without this type of loading, similar results can be obtained with three grams per day for twenty-eight days. During creatine supplementation, your water intake should be at least sixty-four ounces (eight glasses) per day.

8. Bovine Colostrum

Colostrum is a special non-milk breast secretion produced by all mammalian mothers during the first forty-eight hours after they give birth. Colostrum contains special antibodies, immunoglobulins, complex proteins and growth factors capable of triggering at least fifty processes and functions in the newborn. Recently, researchers have discovered that colostrum from bovine sources has many health benefits for adults in general and bodybuilders in particular.

This is because bovine colostrum contains many muscle-building complex proteins and growth factors, including growth hormone. Doctors and other health-care providers have recommended using colostrum for its numerous therapeutic and preventive benefits.

Therapeutic Benefits

- Colostrum growth factors enhance athletic performance naturally by optimizing lean muscle mass while burning excessive fat.
- Its antiviral factors inhibit influenza, herpes, and other viruses.
- Colostrum glycoproteins inhibit *Helicobacter pylori* bacteria, which cause stomach ulcers.
- Interlukin-10, an anti-inflammatory agent found in colostrum, improves arthritis.
- It has effective antibacterial, antifungal, and antiviral effects in the gastrointestinal tract.
- It corrects immunodeficiency by stimulating lymphoid tissue.
- It accelerates wound healing and cartilage repair through various growth factors.
- Colostrum proline-rich polypeptides modulate immunity by activating an underactive immune system through the thymus gland while suppressing an overactive immune system, such as is as seen in autoimmune diseases.
- It is effective against chronic fatigue and leaky gut syndromes.

Preventive Benefits

- Colostrum provides adults with immunization against acute intestinal infections and inflammation.
- It prevents viral and bacterial infections in immunodeficient states.
- It provides safe natural immunity for those at high risk for damage by conventional vaccinations.
- The high concentration of iron-transporting proteins lactoferrin and transferrin in colostrum prevents iron deficiency.
- It is helpful in reducing severity of allergies and infections of all types.
- It prevents some cancers by promoting normal cell growth and DNA synthesis.

Colostrum is effective in the treatment of diverse conditions because it contains proteins, carbohydrates, fat, vitamins and minerals, as well as the antibodies immunoglobulin A and immunoglobulin G in concentrations approximately 100 times higher than in cow's milk. It also contains insulin-like growth factors and insulin-like growth factor I, hormones that can improve athletic performance.

The one potential side effect of using bovine colostrum is a flu-like illness that can start when first using the supplement. This occurs in a small number of people and is just due to an abrupt activation of the immune system. Fever, chills, muscle aches and pains can occur and last several days but then disappear as the system becomes accustomed to colostrum. One can avoid this side effect entirely by starting with very low doses (one capsule per day for four days, then two for four days, etc.) and working up to the maximum dose (usually four to six 500-milligram capsules twice daily on an empty stomach).

Rare, highly sensitive individuals could be allergic to colostrum, but even those with a milk (casein) allergy or lactose intolerance can usually tolerate the supplement without any significant side effects. If you are not sure you should try taking bovine colostrum, check with a naturopath or a doctor familiar with the product.

For more information on colostrum see *Colostrum: Man's First Food, The White Gold Discovery* by Bernard Jensen, PHD (Bernard Jensen Publisher, 1993).

9. Chrysin

Take 500 milligrams twice daily. Chrysin is the chemical name for a type of isoflavone (bioflavonoid) that minimizes the conversion of testosterone to either estrogen or dihyrdotestosterone by blocking an enzyme known as aromatase. Too much estrogen can cause increased fat gain, water retention and breast enlargement in males, while too much dihydrotestosterone can cause prostate enlargement and accelerated male pattern baldness.

Chrysin is often found in various bodybuilding supplements used to boost testosterone levels naturally. It can, however, be used on its own. Chrysin is a naturally occurring chemical extracted from a plant called *Passiflora coerulea*. Several studies conducted on chrysin have shown it to increase natural production and blood levels of testosterone by 30 percent. This means that testosterone levels in the blood could increase without the usual conversion into estrogen or dihydrotestosterone.

10. Tribulus Terrestris

Take 750 to 1,500 milligrams daily in divided doses. Also known as gokhru, nature's Viagra® and puncturevine, tribulus terrestris naturally increases luteinizing hormone, a pituitary hormone that stimulates the manufacture of testosterone. It contains diosgenin and other as yet not fully identified saponins, which are thought to be the active ingredients.

Tribulus can increase your level of testosterone by 30 percent or more within five days and without any clinically proven toxic effects. Since testosterone promotes protein synthesis and positive nitrogen balance, the benefits for the bodybuilder or any athlete are muscle cell growth and increased body strength. In addition it offers faster recuperation and recovery from muscular stress. Tribulus also has a mild diuretic effect, increases muscle size and lean body mass, boosts immunity, lowers cholesterol levels, boosts libido and enhances mood.

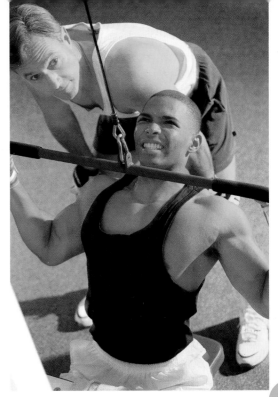

Tribulus increases testosterone, which promotes protein synthesis and positive nitrogen balance.

Other conditions clinically treated with tribulus include:

- anemia
- angina pectoris
- fatigue or neurasthenia
- gonorrhea
- headache
- hepatitis
- indigestion, flatulence, and constipation
- inflammation
- male impotence, low sex drive, and infertility
- painful urination
- psoriasis
- rheumatism
- scabies

No significant adverse effects have been reported with this herb when taken with food. On an empty stomach, it could cause some upset but you can prevent this by eating something with it. Because tribulus can trigger miscarriage, if you are or think you might be pregnant, do not use it; consult your health-care provider.

Other Important Supplements for Bodybuilding

Professional athletes or individuals with frequent or recurrent musculoskeletal injuries due to exercise might wish to take extra supplements both for prevention and to speed healing. Some may be concerned about the adverse effects of increased levels of testosterone in their bodies caused by herbs designed to boost testosterone levels. The best documented nutrients for all these purposes are:

Zinc (30-50 milligrams) is important for optimum growth and muscle metabolism because it is needed by the body to produce testosterone, insulin and growth hormone. It also stimulates the production of the body's primary antioxidant enzyme, superoxide dismutase. Signs of zinc deficiency include hair loss, night blindness not responsive to vitamin A treatment, washboard fingernails and white spots on the nails.

Testosterone is produced in the testes and ovaries and is responsible for the growth of muscles, normal libido and blocking the catabolic (breakdown) effects of cortisol. Without adequate zinc stores, performance can be compromised significantly. Zinc is found in meat, oysters, poultry, eggs, liver and wholegrain bread made with yeast.

Zinc is important for muscle growth.

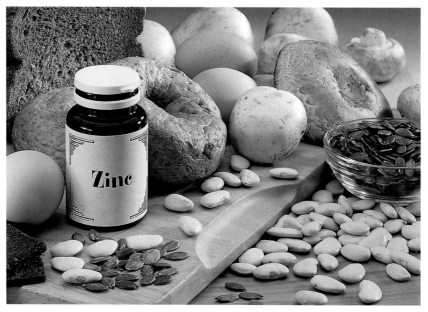

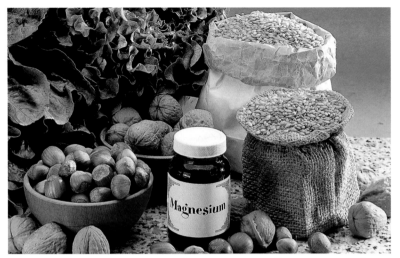

Magnesium (250-400 milligrams) is vitally important for both peak cardiovascular and optimal skeletal muscle function. Regular supplementation prevents muscle spasms, cramps and pain, which is very important for bodybuilders. Magnesium is also a catalyst for calcium absorption, and is part of healthy teeth and bones, where it is stored. Excessive dairy product intake tends to offset magnesium stores in the body. The best food sources are leafy green vegetables; other green foods such as spirulina, chlorella and other algae; whole grains, nuts, and legumes. If you have hard water where you live, this is also a good source of minerals, including magnesium!

Chromium Picolinate (600-800 micrograms) is needed for optimum insulin function, enhanced lean body mass and fat loss. Chromium helps the body use blood sugar and carbohydrates for energy. Strenuous exercise depletes chromium and, unless replenished, fatigue and other low blood sugar reactions such as light-headedness can inhibit optimal performance. There is no evidence that chromium picolinate burns fat or creates more lean body mass. On the other hand, if weight-training programs are not having much of an impact, a chromium deficiency should be suspected. Hair mineral analysis is one way to determine your body's level of this trace mineral. Some good dietary sources of chromium are brewer's yeast, mushrooms, oysters, apples, prunes, nuts, whole grains, meats, cheese, egg yolks, and asparagus.

Supplementation of magnesium prevents muscle spasms, cramps, and pain.

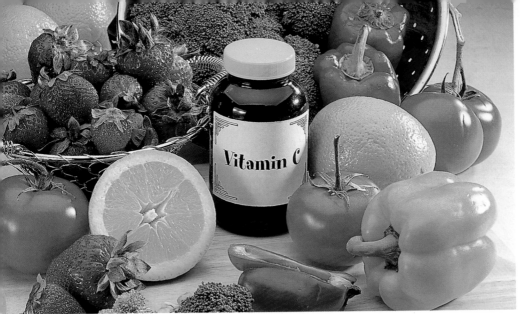

Vitamin C works to both reduce muscle damage and boost strength.

Vitamin C (three grams or more daily, depending on bowel tolerance) has been shown to reduce muscle damage after working out and aid in muscle recuperation by reducing cortisol levels after intense exercise. Growth hormone, testosterone and insulin are all, to various degrees, dependent on an adequate supply of vitamin C. The value of vitamin C as an antioxidant and as a crucial nutrient in bone health are well documented. If you lift weights, vitamin C supplementation can be of noticeable help in boosting strength and stamina while preventing musculoskeletal injuries. It is essential to the development and maintenance of the fat, muscle and bone framework of the body, which is important for gaining strength. It's found in red peppers, broccoli, citrus fruits, tomatoes, and strawberries.

Proanthocyanidins (300 milligrams or more daily) from grape seed extract or pine bark extract are best known as pycnogenols and are one of the bioflavonoids with strong antioxidant protective activity, especially for muscles, ligaments and nervous tissues. It also aids in the absorption of vitamin C. The value of bioflavonoids in preventing exercise damage has been well documented for several decades. For example, in a 1965 study, when citrus bioflavonoids (525 milligrams daily) were administered to professional baseball players, this reduced the overall time lost to injuries by 65 percent and the average recovery time by 54 percent when compared to untreated controls. In addition to being among the most powerful antioxidants, proan-thocyanidins are of great benefit to the heart and circulatory system, which is important during strenuous workouts. (For more information on proanthocyanidins, see *Nature's Best Heart Medicines* by Suzanne Diamond, *alive* Natural Health Guides, 2000).

Methyl-sulfonyl-methane (MSM; 6,000 milligrams or more daily) is a naturally occurring organic source of nutritional sulfur found in ever-diminishing quantities in fresh fruits and vegetables; it is commonly lost during storage and cooking. MSM is a stable metabolite of dimethyl sulfoxide, a substance popularized in the 1970s and 80s for its ability to reverse pain and inflammation in arthritis and other degenerative diseases. Dimethyl sulfoxide can be used to enhance both nutrient and drug absorption into body cells. Unfortunately, the use of dimethyl sulfoxide causes individuals to develop a severe garlic odor to the breath and body. MSM has all the same properties as dimethyl sulfoxide, but is odorless and has no side effects at any dosage.

Sulfur is a critical component of many important amino acids contained in cellular proteins, enzymes, hormones and other body structures. In high doses, MSM is a powerful free-radical scavenger, improves circulation, boosts nutrient absorption, reduces inflammation, and helps reduce the build-up of lactic acid, the chemical causing muscle soreness and fatigue after strenuous exercise. In addition, MSM fights fatigue, helps hair and nails grow faster and has been shown to have antiparasitic properties. The efficacy of MSM is enhanced by vitamin C supplementation. The beneficial effect of glucosamine sulfate in the reversal of osteoarthritis is thought to be related to its sulfur component, something that can be delivered to the body very effectively by MSM. MSM, coupled with an adequate protein intake, also replicates glucosamine sulfate's joint-healing powers.

Coenzyme Q10 (Ubiquinone) (100-200 milligrams daily) is produced in your body and protects against exercise-induced muscle injury and fatigue. It is also important in the conversion of food to energy. Many reports also indicate that coenzyme Q10 is an effective remedy in the treatment of chronic fatigue syndrome and other immune system diseases involving damaged cellular mitochondria. Its value is limited by its high price.

MSM helps reduce the build-up of lactic acid, which causes sore muscles and fatigue after a work out.

Enzymes promote the healing of exercise-damaged tissues.

Proteolytic Enzymes (three or more capsules daily). Trypsin and chymotrypsin, usually considered as enzymes that break down dietary protein in the gastrointestinal tract, also have been shown to promote the healing of many exercise-damaged tissues. Bromelain (from pineapple stalks) and papain (from papayas) have been reported to have similar beneficial effects.

L-carnitine (1,000-2,000 milligrams daily) does not build bigger muscles but has a protective effect against exercise-induced pain and damage. This appears to be primarily related to its vasodilation property, which improves energy metabolism of damaged muscle. Carnitine is therapeutically effective in the treatment of coronary heart disease because normal cardiac function is dependent on adequate concentrations of carnitine in heart muscle. Carnitine helps increase muscle strength and stamina. In the body, carnitine is manufactured from the amino acid lysine and vitamin C.

In addition to its use as an enhancer of athletic performance, carnitine is used to fight the following:
- angina pectoris
- chronic fatigue
- diabetes
- high cholesterol and high triglyceride levels
- hypoglycemia

Carnitine is generally regarded as being very safe—it has even been added to infant formula. It is found in greater amounts in animal-derived foods than in plant-based foods.

Acetyl-L-carnitine (one to two grams before you work out and at bedtime), an L-carnitine derivative, has been shown to reduce the high catabolic cortisol levels in the blood after intense exercise.

Gamma Oryzanol (100-300 milligrams daily) is an extract of rice that lowers cholesterol by decreasing its absorption from the gut, stimulates the release of growth hormone and testosterone, increases strength during resistance training and helps symptoms associated with menopause and aging. It also has antioxidant and fat-mobilizing powers and promotes the release of endorphins, the "feel-good" brain chemicals. While there are no significant side effects, gamma oryzanol can interfere with the results of thyroid lab tests.

Boron (three to six milligrams daily) is generally known for its ability to boost bone density, strength and health. It is also a very effective part of a comprehensive natural regime to help reverse osteoarthritis and as an aid for building muscle and increasing testosterone levels. Some people also use boron for enhancing cognitive function and fine motor skills.

Supplemental boron may also increase estrogen levels in postmenopausal women and healthy men, so it may be a double-edged sword for those wanting to build muscle as opposed to fat, something that is stimulated by higher estrogen levels. Adverse reactions in doses below ten milligrams per day are unlikely and have never been reported by regular users of this supplement. If you use boron regularly, lab tests for estrogen and testosterone would be a good idea.

Ipriflavone (600 milligrams daily with food) is a supplement used to prevent and treat osteoporosis but it can be a useful body-building supplement as well because of its bone-strengthening properties. Ipriflavone is a semisynthetic isoflavone manufactured in the laboratory from daidzein, a compound derived from soy; it also occurs naturally in bee propolis.

More than sixty clinical studies since the 1980s have indicated that long-term treatment with ipriflavone can restore bone density and prevent fractures in elderly patients with established osteoporosis. The average increase in bone density using ipriflavone in addition to calcium is between 1.4 and 2 percent after six months and 5.8 percent after twelve months.

Ipriflavone has a chemical structure similar to that of estrogen but has no estrogenic or other hormonal activity. Ipriflavone can bind to estrogen receptors in bone tissue without exhibiting undesirable estrogenic effects on the breast and uterus. It may therefore be a safer alternative for many women, especially those predisposed to female cancers.

Recently made available in Canadian and American health food stores, ipriflavone has been commonly prescribed in Italy, Hungary and Japan as a mainstream treatment for osteoporosis. Despite being a natural substance, ipriflavone was first registered in Japan in 1988 as a drug, under the name Osten®. In addition to osteoporosis, ipriflavone shows promise in treating other bone disorders, hyperparathyroidism and tinnitus caused by otosclerosis.

Ipriflavone has bone-strengthening properties.

Ipriflavone does the following:

- increases calcium uptake by bone
- inhibits bone breakdown
- enhances bone formation
- builds stronger muscles through its anabolic effects
- enhances protective effects of estrogens on mineral density, without having any direct estrogen-like activity
- reduces bone pain by an average of 45 percent at six months and 62 percent at twelve months
- moves nutrients into building muscle and bone and away from being stored as fat
- increases endurance and stamina naturally
- decreases cholesterol and lowers bad LDL cholesterol while increasing good HDL cholesterol

Ipriflavone has no side effects or toxicity at any dose, but should not be taken by persons using theophylline (an asthma drug) because it may temporarily inhibit liver detoxification pathways, leading to higher than normal levels of theophylline in the blood.

Saw palmetto (*Serenoa repens*) (two grams of whole berries or 320 milligrams of a standardized lipophilic extract) comes from a palm tree native to the southern Atlantic coast and has become popular as a treatment for enlarged prostate in both Europe and the United States.

Saw palmetto extract is not a bodybuilding supplement but it can be used by bodybuilders to offset the side effects of increased levels of testosterone in the body. Testosterone converts in the body to dihydrotestosterone; saw palmetto blocks the enzyme that facilitates that conversion. It is thought that high levels of dihydrotestosterone are at least partially to blame for prostate enlargement and for acne and male pattern baldness in men and women, as well as unwanted facial hair in women.

Stinging Nettle Root (one to two teaspoons of standardized tincture or one 500-milligram capsule twice daily). Bodybuilders can use nettle root, like saw palmetto, for its testosterone-boosting effects as well as its ability to prevent the side effects of excessive testosterone conversion to dihydrotestosterone.

This herb can boost your level of free testosterone, the active form, by blocking the binding of testosterone to its carrier protein. Another natural remedy that can do this is avena sativa, an extract from wild oat straw. Both stinging nettle and avena sativa are also aphrodisiacs because they make more free testosterone available to the body.

The actual level of testosterone production does not generally decrease as men age but the amount of free circulating testosterone decreases as more gets bound to its carrier protein and becomes unavailable for the body's use. Nettle root can reduce the protein (globulin) binding process of testosterone by almost ten-fold.

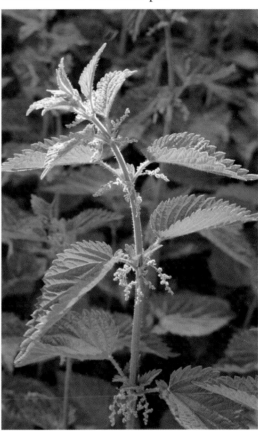

Freeing testosterone through supplementation with nettle root is also effective therapy for benign prostatic hyperplasia. In traditional medicine, stinging nettle root has been used for arthritis and as a diuretic and an astringent. It is thought to work for all these conditions because it contains polysaccharides with immunomodulating and weak anti-inflammatory effects.

Stinging nettle root can boost the level of free testosterone in the body.

Indole-3-Carbinol (100 milligrams twice daily) can deactivate excessive estrogen while enhancing testosterone in the body and thereby prevent fat storage as well as breast cancer and other diseases associated with too much estrogen, including uterine fibroids, endometriosis and ovarian cysts. Indole-3-carbinol is a compound occurring naturally in cruciferous vegetables such as cabbage, broccoli and brussels sprouts. It is a potent defense against excessive estrogen from any source.

You Might Also Have Heard About...

Pyruvate (pyruvic acid; 500-1,000 milligrams three times daily) is created in the body during the metabolism of carbohydrates and protein and has been widely promoted as a weight loss supplement and antioxidant agent. Pyruvate is present in several foods including red apples, cheese, dark beer and red wine. Pyruvate is not an essential nutrient and deficiency of it is not associated with any health problems.

Unfortunately, the studies done on pyruvate are short-term and involved only a small number of individuals. When compared to placebo, pyruvate was found to enhance weight loss and reduce body fat in overweight adults consuming a low-fat diet. Animal studies suggest that pyruvate increases resting metabolic rate. A small number of clinical trials also indicate that pyruvate supplements improve exercise endurance, all useful to the bodybuilder.

When this supplement became available in health-food stores a few years ago, many of my patients, having read the hype, purchased pyruvate supplements. None that I can recall were pleased with the weight-reducing effects. More research or clinical studies should be done before I could recommend the use of this supplement.

Conjugated Linoleic Acid (CLA; two grams three times daily) is a type of fat found in meats and dairy products. Bodybuilders are taking CLA in large doses but there is no objective evidence indicating that it does any good. Animal studies have shown that CLA is capable of reducing body fat, increasing muscle mass, lowering cholesterol, inhibiting cancer growth and preventing or reversing arterial disease. What is uncertain at this time is whether or not CLA works the same way in people.

If you are just beginning a supplement program to complement regular exercise, do not expect instant results. All the nutrients discussed above take time (at least three to six months) to show noticeable improvement since it takes that long to grow the several billion new cells that will incorporate the new influx of nutrients. The best times to take supplements are one hour or so before and immediately following an exercise session and at bedtime. It's a good idea to discuss supplement programs with your health-care provider.

The Best Bodybuilding Diet

While bodybuilding supplements are important, they cannot replace a healthy diet. The best diet is one that provides the body with the raw material it needs for muscle growth.

Fitness experts recommend that you should eat at least one gram of protein for each pound of lean body mass. Lean body mass is something that can be determined for you by skinfold calipers, hydrostatic weighing (weighing under water) or by various electrical impedance devices. Tanita is one brand of weight scales that not only measures your weight, but also your body fat percentage and lean body mass (your weight minus the fat). For example, if you weigh 200 pounds and your body fat percentage is 15 percent, your lean body mass should be 170 pounds. To sustain your present mass, you must consume at least eat 170 grams of protein a day.

To gain more muscle or lean weight, double that intake (340 grams of protein a day). This is provided that you have normal kidney function capable of filtering large amounts of protein. The highest-quality protein can be found in foods such as organic beef, lamb, chicken, turkey, fish, eggs, and skim milk. All of these are fine provided you have no allergies to them.

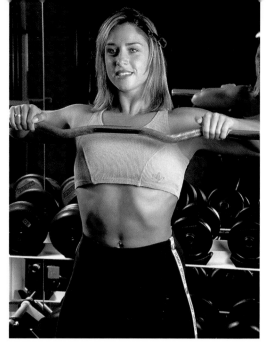

A healthful diet will provide the body with the raw material needed for muscle growth.

Simple carbohydrates (sugar) in any form should be avoided. This includes food items such as pop, candies, cakes, white bread and pasta, sweetened cereals, chips, fried foods, and a long list of junk and fast foods. Whole grains, fruits, vegetables, and legumes (starchy beans) are all acceptable, provided they are well tolerated.

Frequent small meals that contain high-protein foods are ideal.

The only types of high-fat foods that should be eliminated are those containing alcohol, fried food, and junk foods (burgers, fries, ice cream, pastries, croissants, most muffins, doughnuts).

Frequent small meals, every two to three hours, are ideal. If you eat only one or two times a day, your body goes into a "fat conservation mode." Unless you eat often enough, as soon as you do eat, your body will automatically store the food as fat, regardless of the quality

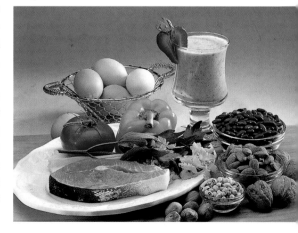

Food Exchange Menu

Exchange List	Recommended	Avoid
Bread and Cereal: Six or more servings per day, whole grains only	•Lentils •Green peas •Beans (dried) •Potatoes with skin •Sweet potatoes •Whole-wheat bread (protein enriched) •Enriched cereals •Enriched whole-wheat pasta	•White-flour products
Fats: Five or more servings per day	•Fish-oil rich foods	•Processed meats and cold cuts
Fruits: Five or more servings per day	•Fresh, frozen or canned fruits, both whole and juice	•Added sugar
Meat and Meat Substitutes: Ten servings per day	•Meats •Poultry •Fish, especially cold-water, oily fish (salmon, herring, mackerel) •Shellfish •Almond, sesame or macadamia butter •Nuts, including pumpkin seeds	•Processed foods
Dairy: Four or more servings per day	•Skim milk •Kefir •Plain yogurt	•Cheeses •Whole or 2% milk •Sweetened dairy products
Vegetables: Three or more servings per day	•Fresh, frozen or canned vegetables, both whole and juice	•None

Note: Include six to eight cups of fluids, such as water, per day.

of that food. Drink at least two liters of water per day and have a relatively larger breakfast to maximally boost metabolism and fat burning enzymes in the body.

Conclusion . . . .

To some extent, we are all building our bodies, regardless of age or sex. Some of us may be doing it better than others and achieving higher degrees of wellness as a direct result. While there is no attempt here to encourage anyone to look like a chiseled, lean, mean fighting machine, the same diet and nutritional supplements that work in combination with strength training exercises for professional bodybuilders will work to enhance wellness for those with more modest physical fitness goals.

Each and every one of the supplements discussed in this book will help anyone lose excess body fat while gaining lean body mass. This is not a weight-loss program. If anything, it is a bodybuilding and fat-loss program, which just about any reasonably healthy person can apply. Here's wishing you much success in looking fitter, feeling better and enjoying greater energy in the years to come.

37

Zoltan Rona

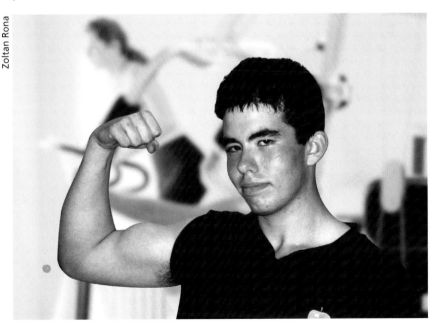

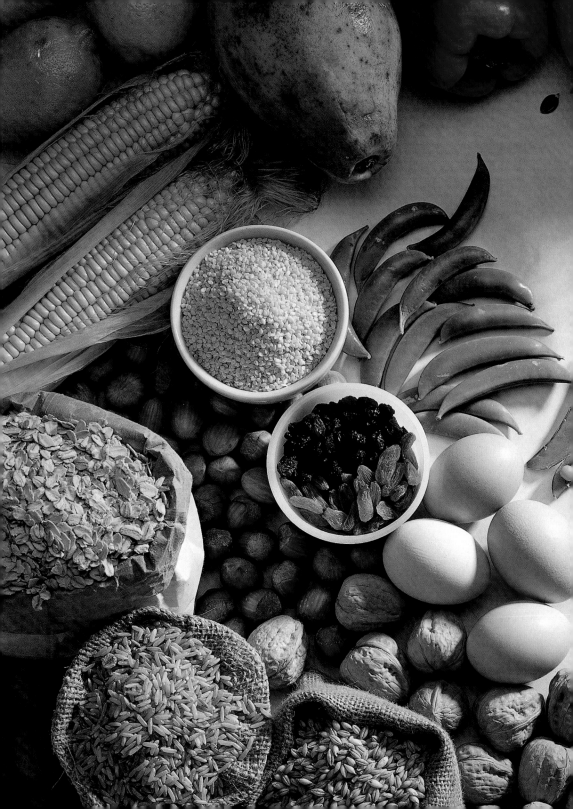

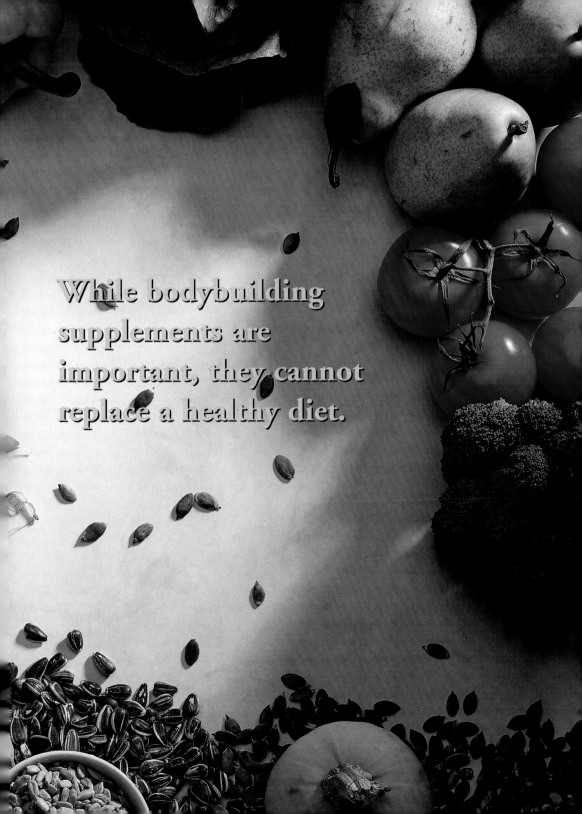

While bodybuilding supplements are important, they cannot replace a healthy diet.

Banana Milkshake

Bananas are rich in minerals, most notably potassium, and contain good amounts of vitamin C.

2 cups (500 ml) **organic whole milk**

3 ripe bananas

1 tbsp unpasteurized honey

1 tsp freshly squeezed lemon juice

Fresh mint, for garnish

Place all ingredients in a blender and blend until smooth.

Serves 2

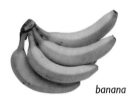

banana

Strawberry Milkshake

Strawberries contain even more minerals than bananas as well as vitamins A, C and B-complex.

2 cups (500 ml) **organic whole milk**

2 cups (500 ml) **strawberries**

1 tbsp unpasteurized honey

1 tsp freshly squeezed lemon juice

Fresh mint, for garnish

Pinch ground cinnamon (optional)

Place all ingredients in a blender and blend until smooth. Sprinkle with cinnamon for extra flavor.

Serves 2

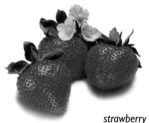

strawberry

Add your favorite protein powder to either of these tasty shakes for a high-protein snack or meal replacement.

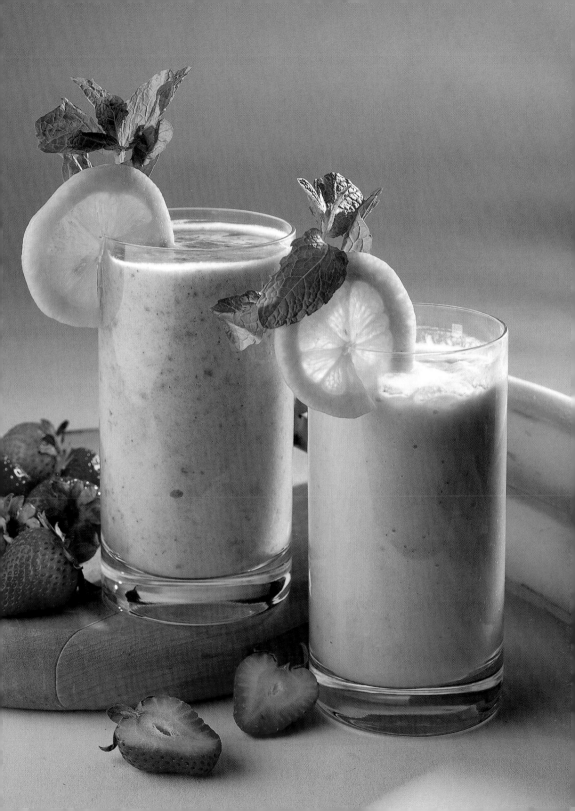

Hercules Breakfast

This power breakfast would make Hercules proud. High in both protein and taste, it is more than satisfying after even the most strenuous work out.

1 large sweet potato, peeled and cut in ½" (1 cm) **cubes**

1 tbsp butter

4 free-range eggs

1 tbsp extra-virgin olive oil

2 cups muesli

1 tbsp unpasteurized honey

2 nectarines, sliced

2 tbsp cashews, roasted and broken into pieces

1 cup (250 ml) **whole milk**

4 slices multigrain bread, toasted

In a pan, heat butter over low heat and sauté the sweet potato until golden brown.

In a separate pan, heat olive oil over low heat then crack the eggs into the pan and cook them until whites and yolks are slightly firm.

In a bowl, combine muesli, honey, and cashews. Pour in milk and place nectarine on top.

Place eggs, sweet potato, and toast on a plate and serve with the muesli and orange juice.

Serves 2

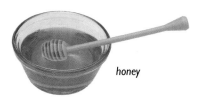

honey

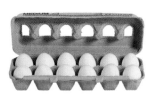

free-range eggs

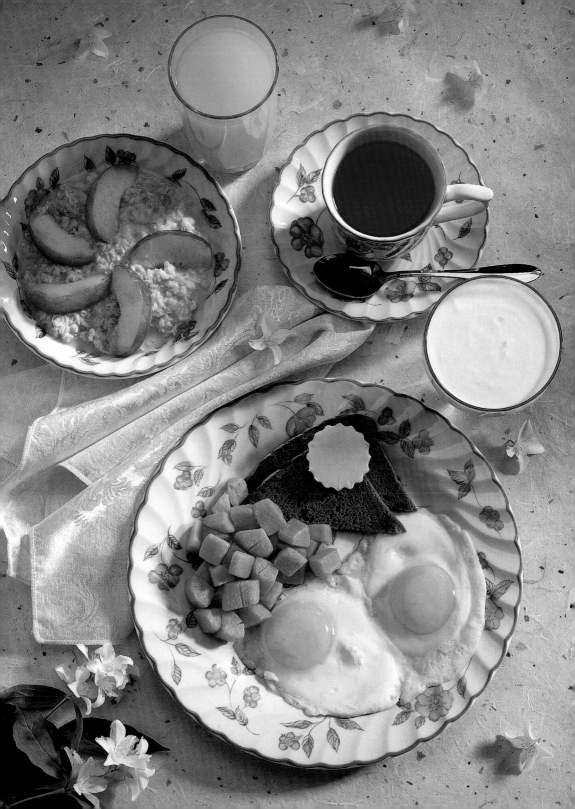

Mung Bean-Vegetable Soup

The mung beans in this recipe will provide a good source of vegetable protein for your daily needs. Remember, an overload of protein (which is often the result of eating meat) causes painful uric acid deposits in the joints.

1 cup (250 g) **mung beans**

3 tbsp extra-virgin olive oil

2 cloves garlic, sliced

1 small white onion, chopped

1 cup (250 g) **green string beans, cut 1"** (2.5 cm) **long**

1 cup (250 g) **carrots, diced**

1 cup (250 g) **celery, diced**

1 cup (250 g) **Brussels sprouts, quartered**

1 cup (250 g) **fresh or frozen corn kernels**

1 cup (250 g) **green peas**

2 ½ cups (375 ml) **vegetable stock or water**

2 bay leaves

Sea salt to taste

2 tsp fresh parsley, chopped, for garnish

Soak the mung beans in water for at least 2 hours. Drain and rinse with fresh water. Drain again.

In a pot, bring 2 cups of water and 1 teaspoon of sea salt to a boil, add the mung beans and cook for 25 to 30 minutes or until tender. Make sure the mung beans are not overcooked otherwise they will burst open.

In a large pan, heat oil over medium heat and sauté garlic and onion, then add carrots, celery, Brussels sprouts, beans, corn, and peas. Stir until translucent. Add vegetable stock, bay leaf, cayenne and salt. Cover and simmer for 10 to 12 minutes. Add the mung beans and gently heat through.

Garnish with parsley and serve.

Serves 2

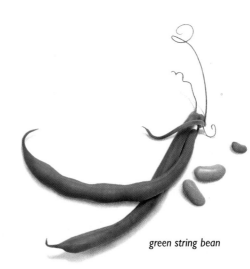

green string bean

44

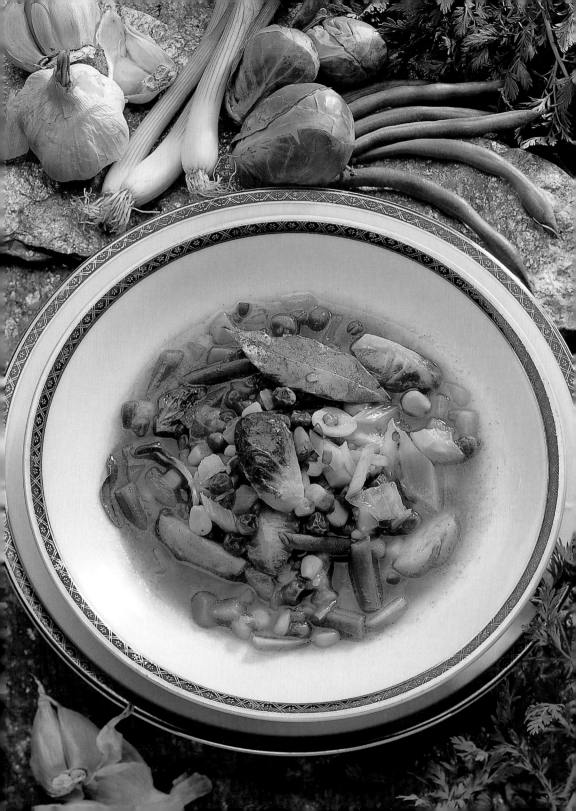

Cabbage-Sprout Salad with Walnuts

Cabbage helps the liver to detoxify as well as supplies antioxidants, vitamin C and beta carotene to fight off free radicals. The walnut provides healthy fats and contains fair amounts of protein, zinc, calcium, and potassium.

1 cup (250 ml) **white cabbage, julienned**

1 cup (250 ml) **red cabbage, julienned**

1 cup (250 ml) **apple, peeled and julienned**

½ cup (125 ml) **walnuts**

½ cup (125 ml) **alfalfa sprouts**

Dressing:

4 tbsp cold-pressed olive or walnut oil

2 tbsp freshly squeezed grape juice

Sea salt and freshly ground pepper, to taste

In a bowl, whisk together all dressing ingredients. Toss cabbage, apple, and walnut with half the dressing. Place onto plates, arrange alfalfa sprouts on top and drizzle with remaining dressing.

Serves 2

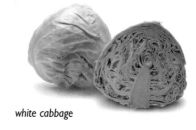

white cabbage

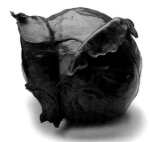

red cabbage

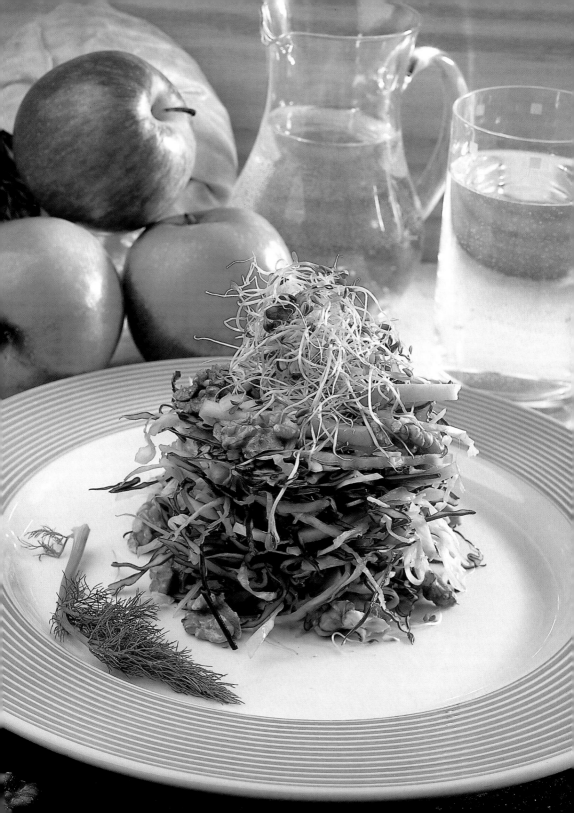

French Salad with Egg and Olives

The vitamin B6 found in greens and carrots aids the absorption of zinc provided by the egg as well as facilitates conversion of healthy oils to prostaglandins.

1 large English cucumber, thinly sliced lengthwise

2 large tomatoes, cut in wedges

2 large carrots, thinly sliced lengthwise

2 cups (500 ml) **organic mixed greens or Romaine lettuce, cut in 1"** (2.5 cm) **strips**

1 small red onion, julienned

¼ cup (60 ml) **black olives**

2 large free-range eggs, soft boiled and sliced

Dressing:

¼ cup (60 ml) **apple cider vinegar**

¼ cup (60 ml) **cold-pressed walnut oil**

1 tbsp fresh tarragon, chopped

1 tbsp Dijon mustard

1 tbsp balsamic vinegar

1 tbsp shallot, minced

1 clove garlic, minced

In a bowl, whisk together all dressing ingredients.

In a large bowl, combine the vegetables and olives. Garnish with the egg then pour the dressing over top and serve.

Serves 2

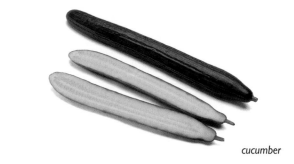

cucumber

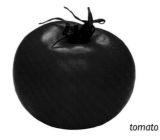

tomato

To soft boil the egg, bring a small pot of water to a boil and slowly add the egg with a large spoon. Cook for exactly 7 minutes then remove from heat, drain the water and rinse the egg under cold water. Crack the top of the egg immediately to prevent the egg from cooking any longer.

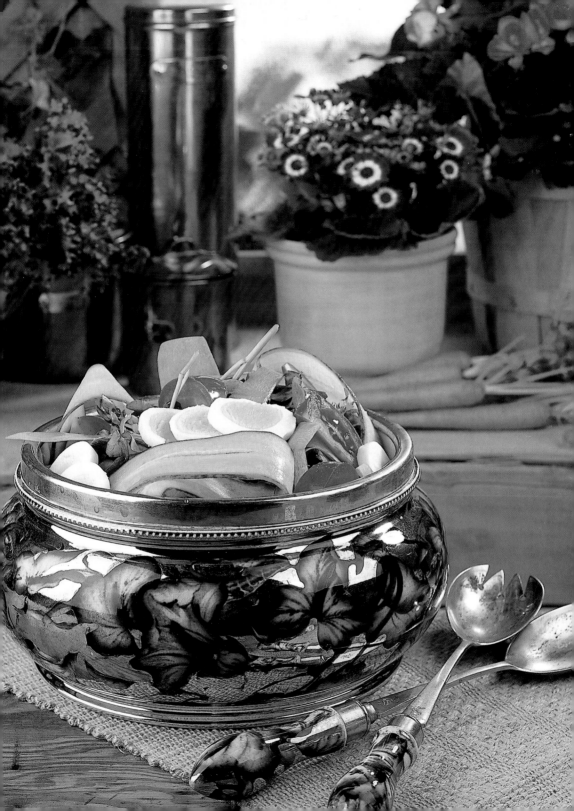

Tuna Sandwich

Of all fish, tuna has the highest proportion of protein and one is of the lowest in fats. Prepared this way, tuna sandwiches will soon become a favorite meal or snack.

2 cans tuna, rinsed and drained

1 large avocado, sliced

½ cup (125 ml) **celery, diced**

½ cup (125 ml) **white onion, diced**

1 tbsp fresh parsley, chopped

½ cup (125 ml) **natural mayonnaise**

1 tsp freshly squeezed lemon juice

Sea salt and freshly ground pepper, to taste

4 slices whole grain bread, toasted

Salad greens and tomato, for garnish

In a bowl, combine tuna, vegetables, mayonnaise, and lemon juice; season with salt and pepper. Assemble the sandwich and slice in half. Garnish with greens and tomato and serve.

Serves 2

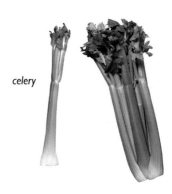

celery

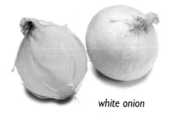

white onion

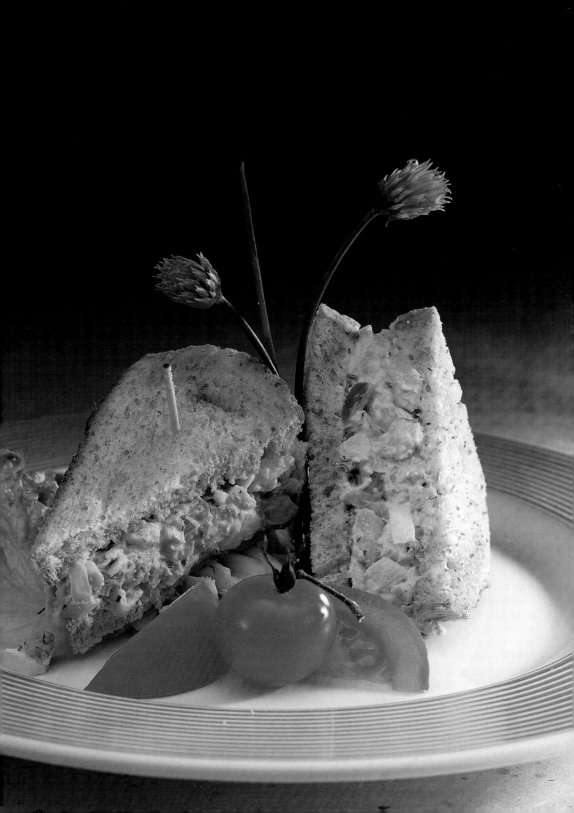

Grilled Vegetable Wrap with Avocado

Tasty and wholesome wraps are easy and fun to assemble and are a big hit with family and friends. I highly recommend the pure taste sensation and maximum nutrition from these simple grilled vegetables.

1 medium zucchini, sliced

1 red bell pepper, cut in 1" (2.5 cm) **wedges**

1 cup (250 ml) **portobello or white mushroom, sliced**

1 tbsp + 4 tbsp extra-virgin olive oil

1 tbsp + ½ tbsp balsamic vinegar

Sea salt and freshly ground pepper, to taste

¼ **cup** (60 ml) **cream cheese**

1 tsp mixed herbs, such as oregano, thyme, and tarragon, chopped

4 leaves green leaf lettuce

2 whole grain tortilla wraps

1 avocado, sliced

2 large tomatoes, cut in wedges

In a pan, heat 1 tablespoon of oil over medium heat and sauté zucchini, pepper, and mushroom (or brush them with oil and roast in oven) until soft and tender. Remove from heat, stir in 1 tablespoon of balsamic vinegar and season with salt and pepper.

In a bowl, combine cream cheese, herbs, and ½ tablespoon of balsamic vinegar then spread mixture on each wrap. Place 2 leaves of lettuce in each wrap then add sautéed vegetables.

To assemble each wrap, fold the bottom 1 ½" (4 cm) over the filling in order to hold everything together, then roll.

Garnish with tomato and avocado slices and serve.

Serves 2

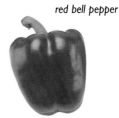

red bell pepper

Putting lettuce leaves on the wrap first prevents the wrap from absorbing too much water and getting soggy.

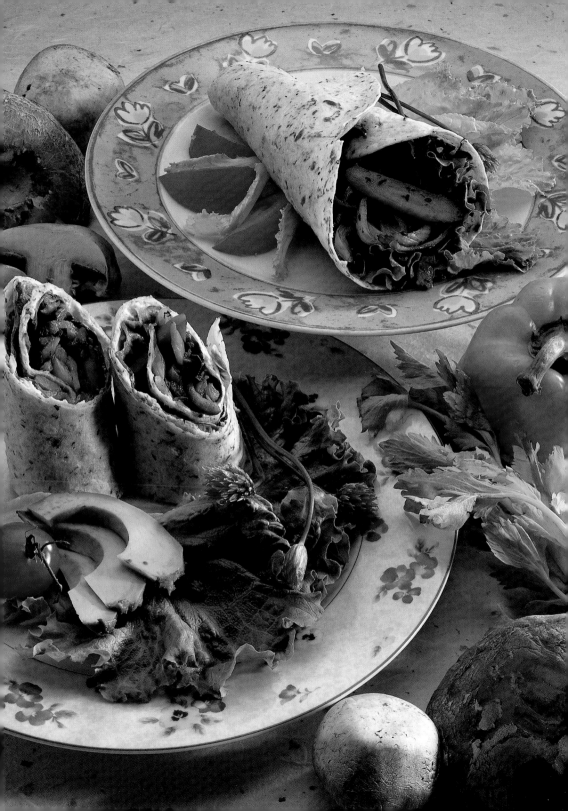

Tuna with Potato Gratin

Simple potato chips (no hydrogenated oil, please) make a wonderful crust for the tuna filets–salt and vinegar flavor is ideal for this recipe. I recommend some lightly blanched asparagus to complete this meal.

Tuna:

2 tuna filets (about ½ lb or 250 g each)

1 cup (250 ml) **potato chips, finely crumbled**

1 tsp lemon juice

1 tsp tarmari

1 tsp ginger, minced

1 tsp garlic, minced

2 tbsp extra-virgin olive oil

Sauce:

¼ cup (60 ml) **tamari**

¼ cup (60 ml) **extra-virgin olive oil**

Sea salt and freshly ground pepper, to taste

Potato Gratin:

3 large russet potatoes, peeled and thinly sliced

1 cup (250 ml) **onion, diced**

½ cup (125 ml) **milk**

½ cup (125 ml) **cream**

1 clove garlic, minced

Pinch nutmeg

Sea salt and freshly ground pepper, to taste

2 tbsp cheese, grated (optional)

Preheat oven to 375°F (190°C).

To prepare the potatoes, butter a loaf pan or casserole dish, place potato on the bottom then sprinkle with onion. In a bowl, combine milk, cream, garlic, nutmeg, and salt and pepper. Pour over potato and sprinkle with your choice of cheese. Bake for 35 minutes on the bottom shelf.

In the meantime, prepare the fish. Crumble the potato chips in a bowl. In a separate bowl, combine lemon juice, tamari, ginger, and garlic. Rub the filets with the lemon juice mixture then dip them in the potato chip crumbs.

In an ovenproof pan, heat oil over medium heat and grill the filets for 2 minutes on each side, then bake in the oven for 5 to 6 minutes or until done. Remove from oven. In a bowl, whisk together the sauce ingredients and pour over the filets.

Serve the tuna immediately with the potato gratin and accompanied with asparagus.

Serves 2

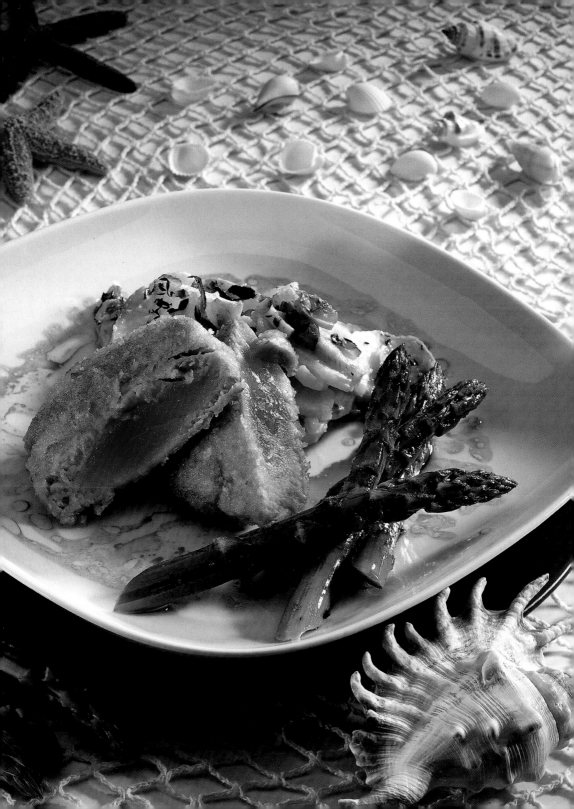

Halibut Filet with Red Beet Salad

Halibut is high in protein yet low in fat. Combined with the red beets and lentils, this dish gives you the nutrients to repair, build, and strengthen the body.

2 halibut filets (about ½ lb or 250 g each)

3 tbsp extra-virgin olive oil

1 tsp freshly squeezed lime or lemon juice

1 tsp garlic, minced

1 tsp ginger, minced

Sea salt and freshly ground pepper, to taste

2 large heads bok choy, leaves separated

Salad:

2 cups (500 ml) **red beets, cooked and diced ½"** (1 cm) **cubes**

1 cup (250 ml) **lentils, cooked**

3 tbsp extra-virgin olive oil

1 tsp freshly squeezed lime or lemon juice

1 tsp honey

1 tsp cilantro, chopped

Sea salt and freshly ground pepper, to taste

Season filet with olive oil, lime or lemon juice, and salt and pepper. Rub the filets on both sides 2 to 3 times with garlic and ginger. Steam for 10 to 15 minutes in a bamboo steamer or double boiler.

In the meantime, bring a pot of salted water to a boil and blanch the bok choy for 3 minutes. Drain and immediately rinse with cold water.

To prepare the salad, whisk together oil, lime juice, honey, and cilantro in a large bowl. Season with salt and pepper. Add warm beets and lentil and toss well.

Place halibut onto plates, arrange bok choy around and serve with the salad.

Serves 2

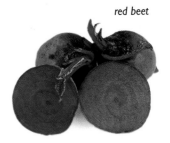

red beet

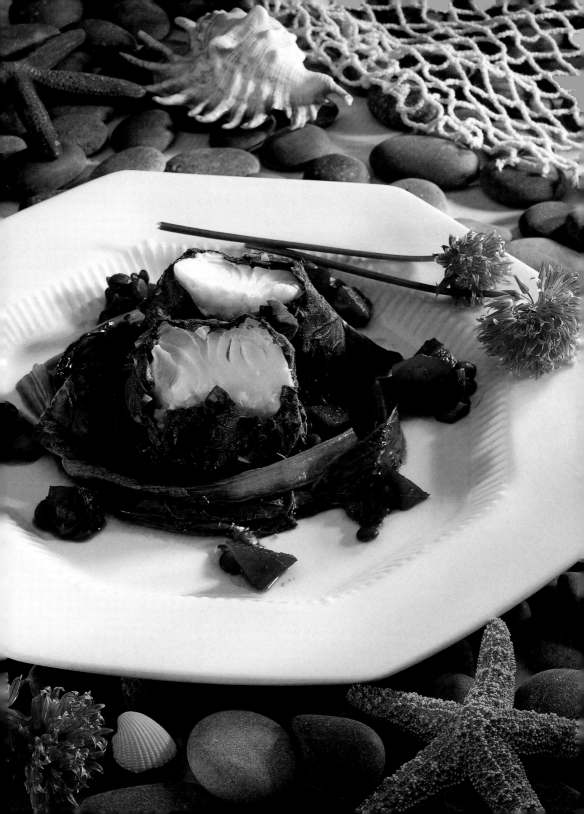

Leek Quiche with Potato Crust

Who says real men don't eat quiche? This muscle-building dish is great for men and women alike. Wonderfully warming and tasty, this quiche has all you need to build strong muscles, providing protein and complex carbohydrates for energy, and the vitamins and minerals needed to utilize protein effectively.

2 large Yukon Gold potatoes, thinly sliced

2 cloves garlic, minced

2 cups (500 ml) **leek, chopped**

1 cup (250 ml) **celery, diced**

½ cup (125 ml) **red bell pepper, diced**

½ cup (125 ml) **yellow bell pepper, diced**

½ cup (125 ml) **green onion, diced**

1 tsp parsley, chopped

1 tsp sage, chopped

3 tbsp extra-virgin olive oil

6 free-range eggs

½ cup (125 ml) **cream**

Pinch ground nutmeg

Sea salt and freshly ground pepper, to taste

1 cup (250 ml) **Gruyère cheese**

Butter, to grease

Preheat oven to 375°F (190°C). Grease a springform pan with butter.

Arrange half the potato slices to cover the bottom of the springform pan and set aside.

In a pan, heat oil over medium heat and sauté all vegetables and herbs until soft and tender. Cool the vegetables to almost room temperature.

In a bowl, beat together egg, cream, nutmeg, salt and pepper. Stir in half the cheese then add the sautéed vegetables and mix well. Pour the mixture over the potato in the springform pan.

Bake on the top shelf of the oven for 10 minutes or until almost solid. Remove from the oven, sprinkle with remaining cheese and place remaining potato slices on top. Bake for 15 minutes longer or until potato is golden brown and fully cooked.

Serve warm with a tomato salad.

Makes 1 quiche

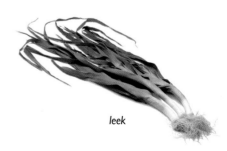

leek

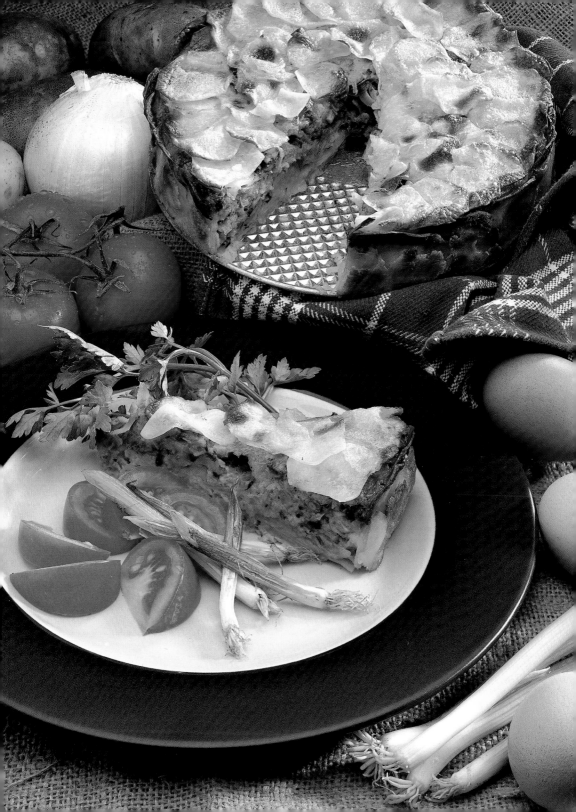

Eggplant with Whole Wheat Spaghetti

Aside from the healthful benefits, this wholesome and hearty vegetarian meal is a snap to make and a favorite to enjoy. Eggplant enhances immunity and inhibits the rise of blood cholesterol induced by fatty foods. And, it's easy to benefit from whole grains with so many whole wheat pastas on the market today.

1 large eggplant, cut in ½" (1 cm) slices

Sea salt and freshly ground pepper

½ cup whole wheat flour

1 free-range egg

1 tbsp cold water

1 cup (250 g) whole wheat bread crumbs

¼ cup (60 g) sesame seeds

½ cup (125 ml) coconut or extra-virgin olive oil

½ lb (225 g) whole wheat spaghetti

1 cup (250 ml) tomato sauce

Season both sides of the eggplant with sea salt and freshly ground pepper. Put the whole wheat flour in a bowl. In another bowl beat the egg with the water. And put the whole wheat bread crumbs and sesame seeds in a third bowl. (You are setting up a sort of production line for breading the eggplant.) Press both sides of an eggplant slice in the whole wheat flour to coat, dip both sides of the slice in egg bowl, then into the bread crumb and sesame seed bowl for a final coating. Repeat with all slices.

In a cast-iron frying pan, heat the oil over medium heat. Brown both sides of the coated eggplant slices. Remove from heat and place in a warm oven at 280°F (130°C) until your pasta and sauce are ready.

Serves 2

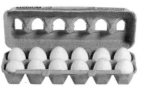

free-range eggs

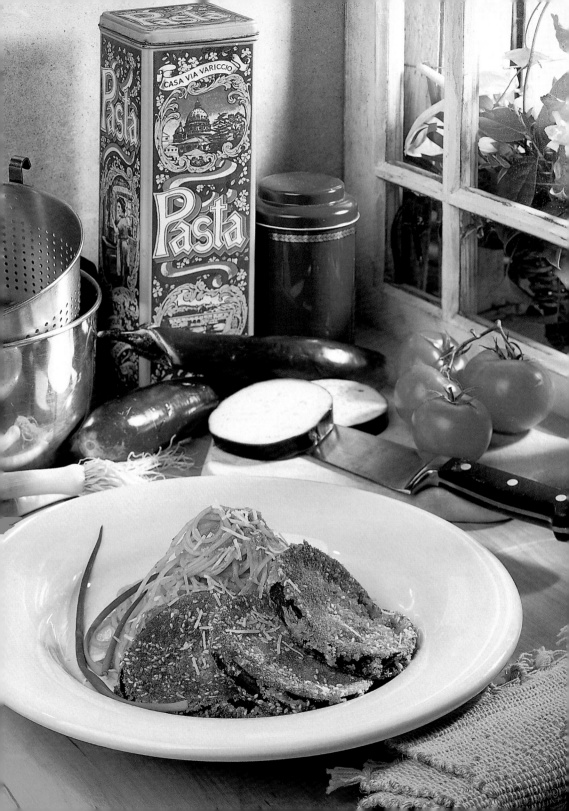

references

Balsom, P. et al. *Sports Medicine*. 18 (1994): 268-80.

Braverman, Eric R. and Carl C. Pfeiffer. *The Healing Nutrients Within*, 2nd ed. Keats Publishing, 1997.

Burke, Edmund R. and Daniel Gastelu, eds. *Avery's Sports Nutrition Almanac*. Garden City Park, NY: Avery Publishing Group, 1999.

Chaitow, Leon. *Amino Acids in Therapy; A Guide to the Therapeutic Application of Protein Constituents*. Thorson's Publishers, 1985.

Graham, A.S. and R.C. Hatton. "Creatine: A Review of Efficacy and Safety." *Journal of the American Pharmacology Assocociation*. 39 (1999): 803-10.

Heinerman, John. *Dr. Heinerman's Encyclopedia of Anti-Aging Remedies*. Paramus: Prentice Hall, 1997, pp. 85-86.

Ivy, J.L. et al. "Effects of Pyruvate on the Metabolism and Insulin Resistance of Obese Zucker Rats." *American Journal of Clinical Nutrition*. 59 (1994): 331-37.

Koshy, K.M. et al. "Interstitial Nephritis in a Patient Taking Creatine." *New England Journal of Medicine*. Vol. 340, no. 10 (1999): 814-15.

Kreider, R.B. et al. "Effects of Creatine Supplementation on Body Composition, Strength, and Sprint Performance." *Medical Science in Sports and Exercise*. Vol. 30, no. 1 (1998): 73-82.

Murray, Michael T. *Encyclopedia of Nutritional Supplements*. Rocklin, CA: Prima Publishing, 1996.

Ode, P. *The Complete Medicinal Herbal*. New York: Dorling Kindersley, 1993, p. 40.

Pearson, D. and S. Shaw. *Life Extension: A Practical Scientific Approach*. New York: Warner Books, 1982.

Poortmans, J.R. and M. Francaux. "Long-Term Oral Creatine Supplementation Does Not Impair Renal Function in Healthy Athletes." *Medical Science in Sports and Exercise*. 31 (1999): 1108-10.

Rona, Zoltan. "Bovine Colostrum Emerges as Immune System Modulator." *American Journal of Natural Medicine*. (March 1998): 19-23.

--- and Jeanne Marie Martin. *Return to the Joy of Health*. Vancouver: alive books, 1995.

Rudman, Daniel. "Growth Hormone, Body Composition, and Aging." *Journal of the American Geriatrics Society*. 33 (1985): 800-7.

Shimomura, Y. et al. "Protective Effect of Coenzyme Q10 on Exercise-Induced Muscular Injury." *Biochemical and Biophysical Research Communications*. Vol. 176, no. 1 (1991): 349-55.

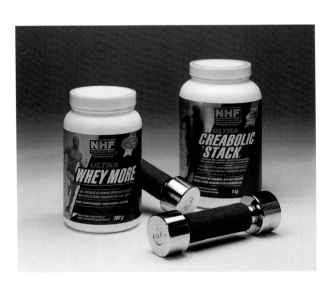

references

Stanko, R.T., et al. "Pyruvate Supplementation of a Low-Cholesterol, Low-Fat Diet: Effects on Plasma Lipid Concentration and Body Composition in Hyperlipidemic Patients." *American Journal of Clinical Nutrition.* 59 (1994): 423-27.

Stanko, R.T. et al. "Enhanced Leg Exercise Endurance With a High-Carbohydrate Diet and Dihydroxyacetone and Pyruvate." *Journal of Applied Physiology.* Vol. 69, no. 5 (1990): 1651-56.

---. "Enhancement of Arm Exercise Endurance Capacity with Dihydroxyacetone and Pyruvate." *Journal of Applied Physiology.* Vol. 68, no. 1 (1990): 119-24.

---. "Body Composition, Energy Utilization, and Nitrogen Metabolism With a 4.25-MJ/d Low-Energy Diet Supplemented With Pyruvate." *American Journal of Clinical Nutrition.* Vol. 56, no. 4 (1992): 630-35.

Tanny, Mandy. *Bodybuilding Nutrition.* New York: HarperPerennial, 1991.

Tarnopolsky, M. and J. Martin. "Creatine Monohydrate Increases Strength in Patients With Neuromuscular Disease." *Neurology.* 52 (1999): 854-57.

Vandenberghe, K. et al. "Long-Term Creatine Intake is Beneficial to Muscle Performance During Resistance Training." *Journal of Applied Physiology.* Vol. 83, no. 6 (1997): 2055-63.

Zuschlag, J.M. "Double-Blind Clinical Study Using Certain Proteolytic Enzyme Mixtures in Karate Fighters. Working Paper." *Mucos Pharma* (1988): 1-5.

First published in 2000 by
alive **books**
7436 Fraser Park Drive
Burnaby BC V5J 5B9
(604) 435–1919
1-800–661–0303

© 2000 by *alive* books

All rights reserved. No part of this book may be reproduced or transmitted in any form or by any means, electronic or mechanical, including photocopying, recording and any information storage and retrieval system, without the written permission of the publisher and the author.

Book Design:
 Liza Novecoski
Artwork:
 Terence Yeung
 Raymond Cheung
Food Styling/Recipe Development:
 Fred Edrissi
Photography:
 Edmond Fong (recipe photos)
Photo Editing:
 Sabine Edrissi-Bredenbrock
Editing:
 Sandra Tonn
 Donna Dawson

Canadian Cataloguing in
Publication Data

Rona, Zoltan MD MSC
 Supplements for Natural Body
 Building

(*alive* natural health guides, 19
ISSN 1490-6503)
ISBN 1-55312-021-3

Printed in Canada

Series 1

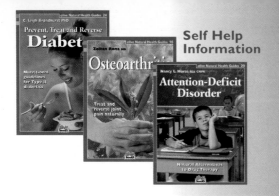

Prevent, Treat and Reverse
Diabet
Nutritional guidelines for Type II diabetics

Osteoarth...
Treat and reverse joint pain naturally

Self Help Information

Attention-Deficit Disorder
Natural Alternatives to Drug Therapy

Series 2

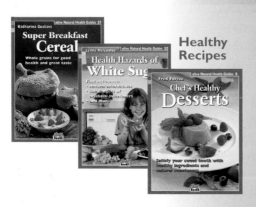

Super Breakfast
Cereal
Whole grains for good health and great taste

Health Hazards of
White Sug...
Find out about:
• natural substitutes and
• the dangers of artificial sweeteners
• and more

Healthy Recipes

Chef's Healthy
Desserts
Satisfy your sweet tooth with healthy ingredients and natural sweeteners

Series 3

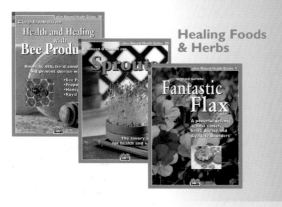

Health and Healing with
Bee Produ...
Boost health, treat cond... and prevent disease w...
• Bee P...
• Propo...
• Honey
• Royal...

Sprou...
The savory s... for health and v...

Healing Foods & Herbs

Fantastic Flax
A powerful defense against cancer, heart disease and digestive disorders

Series 4

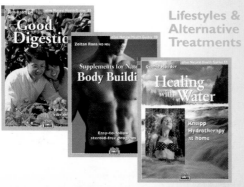

Good Digestio...
Your k... Vibra...

Supplements for Natu...
Body Buildi...
Easy-to-follow steroid-free program

Lifestyles & Alternative Treatments

Healing with Water
Kneipp Hydrotherapy at home

Revolutionary
Health Books

alive **Natural Health Guides**

Each 64-page book focuses on a single subject, is written in easy-to-understand language and lavishly illustrated with full color photographs.

Great gifts at an amazingly affordable price
$9.95

***alive* Natural Health Gui...**
available
at health food stores and nutrition centers

To find a store near you go to **www.alivepublishing...** or call **1-800-663-6580**

alive books
Vancouver
Canada